Hans Georg Brecklinghaus

Rolfing®
Structural Integration

What it achieves, how it works
and whom it helps.

On the author

Hans Georg Brecklinghaus was born 1951. He has a degree in Pedagogy and is a Certified Advanced Rolfer and Rolf Movement Practitioner. He lives in Freiburg, Germany and has been working as practitioner of the Rolfing® method of Structural Integration since 1983.

He has also written a book about body structure and the conception of the human being in the art of ancient Egypt and various essays for professional journals.

Address:

Hans Georg Brecklinghaus
Stadtstrasse 9 a
79104 Freiburg
Germany
Tel.: 0049-761-286866
e-mail: hgbreck@compuserve.de
www.rolfing-praxis.de

Hans Georg Brecklinghaus

Rolfing®

Structural Integration

What it achieves,
how it works and
whom it helps.

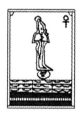

Lebenshaus   Verlag

Rolfing – Structural Integration.
What it achieves, how it works and whom it helps
© 2001 by Hans Georg Brecklinghaus.

American edition, 2002

Published by
Lebenshaus Verlag
Sonnhalde 101
79194 Gundelfingen
Germany

Translated into American
by Simone Lukas-Jogl

Printed by
Lightning® Source Inc., La Vergne, TN

ISBN 3-932803-03-5

Table of Contents

Introduction

Whether you are looking for an "alternative", holistic method to improve your health or want to realize your full human potential, you are nowadays faced with an overwhelming variety of therapies and schools of movement education. Even professionals in the field are having more and more difficulty finding their way around the host of available systems that claim to provide a complementary or alternative method to the traditional ways of medicine or psychology.

As a non-health professional, you are probably concerned with three things: 1) What do I want to achieve for myself? Which problems am I trying to solve? The answer to this personal assessment directly leads to the second question: 2) Which therapy/method would fit my goals? Does it appeal to me? And last, but not least: 3) Is it a well-founded method? Are its practitioners qualified and well-trained?

The book you are looking at is going to introduce you to Rolfing® Structural Integration. Rolfing gets its name from Dr. Ida Rolf, who developed the method. The purpose of Rolfing is to improve the body-structure, the three-dimensional shape of the body, in such a way that the individual person can develop more freely and easily. It strives to help the organism find a natural balance.

Let me elaborate this very general description by giving you a few of the basic assumptions Rolfing is based on:

1. Emotional and physical well-being are dependent on a body-structure that is at ease with gravity.
2. Most people are forced to fight gravity because their body-structures have been thrown more or less off balance.
3. The shapes of our bodies are malleable. Therefore, an organism can be brought (back) to a state of harmonious equilibrium with gravity by a specific kind of connective tissue and muscles manipulation.
4. Rolfing changes the spatial relations among body-parts and so allows gravity to effortlessly align and uplift the structure.
5. The Rolfing process encourages greater somatic awareness. The body is viewed as an expression of the whole being.
6. Core uplift and a body-structure that is both flexible and strong are prerequisites for physical and mental dynamic balance. Rolfing is a way to achieve this.

Rolfing has been around for a few decades. It has proven itself effective in various contexts that call for somatic or emotional work. Among these are: preventive health care, relieving chronic muscular tension, working with structural and postural problems, expanding movement possibilities, enhancing somatic awareness and expression, decreasing chronic stress, preparing for birth, supporting the healing process in chronic joint problems, and many more.

The size of this book requires me to confine myself to essentials. I will provide concise descriptions and lots of practical examples to illustrate the merits as well as the limitations of Rolfing.

My deep respect and gratitude belongs to *Dr. Ida Rolf* who's legacy we took on as practicioners of the method she developed. I also want to appreciate my teachers for what I have learned from them. I feel a debt of gratitude particularly to *Hans Flury*, *Hubert Godard*, *Peter Levine*, *Peter Melchior*, *Carlos Repetto*, *Michael Salveson*, *Robert Schleip* and *Jan Sultan*.

1. The Concept of Rolfing - Structural Integration

a. Basics

The theory of Rolfing deals with four factors, which interrelate and influence each other. They are: structural organization of the human body, gravity, the body's plasticity, and connective tissue.

We all know that the structure of a building determines its stability. The Leaning Tower of Pisa can lean only as long as it does not exceed a certain critical angle. If its foundations sag more, it will eventually topple. A crooked tree is in a somewhat better position; it can change the direction in which it grows and thus adapt to gravity. Have you ever given a thought to how the human body structure achieves or loses stability?

The human body is subject to the influence of gravity just like any other three-dimensional structure. However, we are rarely aware of this simple, but fundamental fact since gravity is energy that we neither see nor hear, smell nor touch.

Perhaps you know someone with a shorter leg. If you take a closer look, you may be able to see that this person's spine has bent to the other side in order to compensate for the uneven support. After all, the body's weight cannot be distributed evenly on uneven legs. The elderly lady with the hunched back, who passed you in the street the other day, has the same problem: She has to constantly struggle with gravity to be able to stand upright.

Extreme examples like these help us realize what is true for everybody: No matter what we are doing, whether we are moving, standing or sitting, we must deal with gravity. In fact, we are constantly dealing with it. Usually, we do that unconsciously with subtle changes of posture. We are never really still. Instead, we oscillate between slightly varying positions. Adapting to the demands of gravity can be a more or less successful, more or less economical enterprise, depending upon the degree of balance we have attained in our body-structures.

Do you remember stacking up building blocks when you were a kid? You quickly discovered how to stack the blocks so that the pile would not collapse. You also realized that the more precisely you put the blocks right on top of each other, the more stable the stack was going to be. And as you were a curious little person, you tested how far the individual blocks could be off the centerline of the pile without crashing it.

The simple example of a pile of building blocks illustrates some of the major characteristics of structural stability: If the centers of gravity in all the blocks are precisely aligned on top of each other, the resulting structure will be stable and perfectly balanced. The organizational pattern of the structure, which is created by the spatial relations of the individual blocks (segments) with each other, is closely linked with gravity: A structure can only remain erect if its organizational pattern takes gravity into account.

But gravity can not only destroy the pile, it is essential to stacking it in the first place: the weight of the blocks is needed to create the counterpressure from the ground which will support the stack. This happens most efficiently when all the individual blocks' centers of gravity can be connected with an invisible vertical line. Another essential prerequisite for a stable stack is that all connecting planes are horizontal.

Since the human body is also a three-dimensional structure in space, we can use the analogy of the block-model very nicely. In the human body, the individual segments would be: head, neck, shoulder girdle, chest, belly, pelvis, thighs, legs and feet.

If the segments of the body are well aligned, their centers of gravity all converge on an imaginary central line. If this line coincides with the plumbline of gravity, the weight of the body is transmitted vertically down to the ground and creates counterpressure upwards. This will support and uplift the individual segments (antigravitation factor). Thus, the organism needs to expend only comparatively little energy to keep itself upright.

You can easily check how well someone's particular structural organization promotes balance in the whole: If you look at their body from the side and imagine a vertical line through the middle, ideally, the following checkpoints should be very *close* to that line: ear, shoulder-joint, elbow, hip joint, knee and ankle. (Fig. 1, right hand picture)

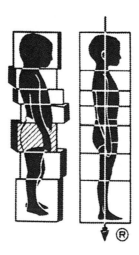

Fig. 1 Unfavorable body structure (left) and more economical body-structure (right)

If the segments of the human structure are, however, shifted, their centers of gravity are taken away from the plumbline and the organism must expend energy to stay upright.

Segments can be *shifted* horizontally to the front, back or sides (see Fig. 1, on the left and Fig. 2). Furthermore, they can be *rotated* around all or any of the three dimensional axes in space. Fig. 1 (left hand picture) demonstrates rotations around the vertical axis. Moreover, the pelvis in this picture is *tilted* forward (rotation around the horizontal side-to-side axis).

Fig. 2 shows rotations around the horizontal front-to-back axis. The pelvis of the woman, for example, is higher on her right side than on her left side. This is

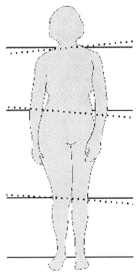

Fig. 2

compensated by a opposite tilt of her shoulders. A structure that is thus off balance must continuously fight gravity, which puts stress on the joints and tends to wear them out. Note also that the relative positions of all the segments are interrelated: the spatial situation of one segment will invariably affect all the others. We will see examples demonstrating this fact later in this book.

What determines the shape of the human body?

If you look at anatomy or physiology textbooks, you will find an elaborate version of something like this: The structure of the human "movement-apparatus" consists of the skeletal bones and muscles. The bones are the static element and provide support for the structure. They determine the basic shape of the human organism. The muscles are the motion element of the body. They cross the joints between the bones and contract to produce movement in the limbs. Descriptions of the fascial web are seldom included, despite the fact that the connective tissue actually constitutes the "organ of form".

Imagine for a moment that you could remove all the intestines, organs, bones, muscles, in short, all the tissues except the connective tissue from your body. What would you see if you looked in the mirror? You would see exactly the shape of your body, its contours down to even the slightest detail, in the form of a three-dimensional network of connective tissue.

All types of connective tissue - the superficial fascial "bodysuit", the fascial sheaths wrapping all the muscles (fascia), the tendons, the ligaments, the fascial envelopes around organs, nerves, and blood vessels - not only connect parts, as implied by the name, they also differentiate between various structures. In this way, connective tissue creates spaces in the body.

The outermost connective tissue layer is called the superficial fascia. It wraps the entire body like one continuous body suit. Each individual muscle, as well as single muscle fibers and bundles of muscle fibers are wrapped in connective tissue bags. These bags are called fascia (Fig. 3) and are continuous with tendons and ligaments. In this way, the fascial system comprises a

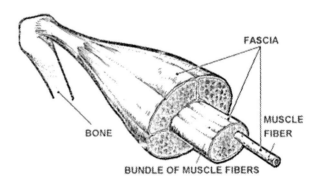

Fig. 3

network of several superficial and deep layers. Since they all hang together, the fasciae allow tensional forces to be transmitted across several body-segments. Furthermore, the fascial wrappings of individual muscles determine how smoothly neighboring muscles can glide alongside or across each other. Moreover, the relative positions of the bones are determined by an intricate interplay of the various tensional forces of surrounding muscles and fasciae.

When traditional anatomy textbooks describe the "movement apparatus", they tend to focus too much on the skeleton as the fundamental static element that keeps the human body upright. I would like to contrast that image with another, which is equally exaggerated but describes functional reality better.

Let us picture the skeletal bones as floating in a mobile environment of muscles, tendons, fasciae, and enveloped organs. This environment of flexible tensional elements determines how and in which directions the bones can move. The bones play only the part of the compressive elements in a tension-compression system. If you imagine a tent, you will immediately understand the image. Without the tent poles, the tent would of course collapse. It could not create any inside space. However, the position of the poles is determined and limited by the tensional pull of the fabric and ropes.

How can a body structure change?

When you observe people standing or walking, you will find that everybody moves differently; everybody has their own pattern of movement which is characteristic of them. However, most of us are not consciously aware of our movement pattern just as we are not normally aware of idiosyncratic behaviors. The various individual ways of holding ourselves upright and moving are first and foremost a product and an expression of our various individual life stories.

Let us start, though, with making a distinction between *posture* and *structure*. Posture, on the one hand, is voluntary; we can change and modify it whenever we choose. Structure, on the other hand, is not usually accessible to voluntary control. Therefore, it is completely useless to remind a child with a collapsed chest to "Stand up straight!" The child may be able to improve her posture for a few minutes. However, she will soon fall back into her usual slouch, because that is her structure and she cannot change her structure by simply making the effort. Habitual "good posture" does not come from holding oneself upright. It happens naturally when a body is free of structural limitations. Then the child is able to stand upright easily and gracefully.

The experiences we make in a lifetime shape our body structures and affect how we move. Whatever life confronts us with emotionally or physically will leave an impact on our previous body structure. In this way, every new factor gets superimposed on the existing pattern and reacts with what is already there. Over time, elements of our personal history and environment blend with our reactions to them and form a complex, individual body structure.

Slight alterations in the static equilibrium of the body can over time develop into major structural flaws, with far-reaching effects on the available postural and movement possibilities. Emotional trauma, injury, invasive medical procedures, disease, and cultural habits can result in structural fixations and a limited scope of movement patterns. Let's have look at two examples.

Susan suffers a sports injury to her right hip joint. Trying to give the painful side a break, she relies on the left half of her body more. The added strain causes the fasciae on the left side of the pelvis and the left leg to thicken and shorten; the muscles that are wrapped in them become less flexible. This produces uneven tensional forces within the tissues which further exaggerate the existing differences. Several segments of Susan's body are being pulled out of vertical alignment as her body tries to compensate for shortness in the left hip.

Your body will compensate to keep you on two legs. Compensations are necessary to maintain as much basic structural stability as possible. Usually they involve areas far away from the original shortness. A very common place for compensations to occur is along the spine. Furthermore, gravity will always tend to amplify structural imbalances.

Joe has a hard time at school and at home. He learns to better be on his guard. For him, life means fighting for what you want and need. His posture reflects that: he is pushing his chest forward aggressively while retracting his shoulders. Although his posture is determined by an emotional rather than a physical condition, it will manifest itself in his body structure just the same as soon as the muscles around the thoracic spine and between the shoulder blades have become chronically tense. The myofasciae (muscles and their fasciae) of the upper back will shorten and thicken. Other parts of the body will structurally adapt. Joe may develop a swayback, for example, and overly straight knees.

But whatever the origins of structural imbalances, unfortunately the loss of structural order and economical motion is not the only problem: Tissues tend to form adhesions if they do not move properly. Wherever layers of tissue are glued together or thickened, the metabolism in the surrounding area will be impaired. Moreover, a chronically tense body will impede sensation as well as emotional flexibility. The autonomic nervous system will be recalibrated to match the constant tissue hypertension. Breathing will not be free and organ function will suffer. Just imagine what a permanently collapsed chest looks like and try to imitate that. Can you feel how difficult it is to breathe?

If your body structure changes, so will the way you move (and the other way around). Structure and movement affect each other. Your body structure develops according to what you do in your life, according to how much and in what ways you move. At the same time, you can only move within the structural limits of your body and your joints.

For example, think of a knee joint. If you walk with a slight swerve of the knee for years, using the hinge joint as if it were a saddle joint, the muscles, tendons, ligaments and menisci in and around your knee will adapt in tension and form. The shape of your knee will change to better fit the asymmetrical use you are putting it to. However, since your body is not designed for it, that will put the knee joints under even more stress and tend to wear them out faster.

I have explained how, because of the plasticity of connective tissue, your body's structure can become less balanced and less stable. By the same token, though, there must be a way to use connective tissue plasticity to bring about greater balance as well. Biochemist *Dr. Ida Rolf* discovered just that. Her great accomplishment was to make a connection between body structure, gravity, connective tissue and body plasticity. In a lifetime of practical application, she developed an equally "simple" and brilliant method to balance body structures in gravity and allow them to align and uplift.

b. Goals of Rolfing

Despite the fact that Rolfing can promote much more than mere physical change, a Rolfer is first and foremost concerned with body structure. The overall goal of Rolfing is to reorganize body structure to move harmoniously with gravity. This goal can be broken down to the following objectives:

1. Establishing the Line: Segments of the body should be organized around an imaginary inner line which in standing comes as close to the vertical plumbline as possible. This inner line starts at the top of the head and connects downwards in front of the spine, through the pelvic floor, between the knees and ankles to the ground. The line is a principle of organization for our bodies. All movements can start from the line and return to it. When you flex to pick something up, for example, your inner line should flex in a balanced way, which will allow the centers of gravity of individual body segments to stay as close to the vertical as possible (Fig. 4, p. 18).

2. Establishing optimum balance between front and back of the body (Fig. 1, p. 7 and Fig. 4, p. 18).

3. To minimize the effort necessary for a particular movement, it should initiated with a reduction of

tone in the antagonists and in the body at large. Namely via stretching of the fascia of the muscles the potential energy, accumulated in the fascia, can be converted into kinetic energy. Moreover, after this initiation, movement should be performed primarily by the deep, intrinsic muscles. The more superficial, extrinsic muscles should only kick in later.

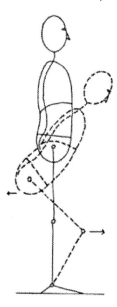

Fig. 4 Folding

In this way, movement will start from the center of the body and translate into arms and legs. The torso as well as the limbs will tend to elongate rather than shorten. We call this the *extension mode* of motion.

Movement of this quality is always two-directional: it includes a settling down from the body center to where the overall motion starts (this is usually the direction of gravity) and the visible movement into the intended direction.

For instance, consider bending forward (Fig. 4, p.18): If your extensor muscles in the front (abdominals) and in the back (hamstrings and back muscles) are free to lengthen, your trunk will remain long and your core unrestricted.

4. Balancing the tone of flexor and extensor muscles of the body (agonists and antagonists): Optimal economy of muscle effort is only possible if flexors and extensors cooperate instead of counteracting each other. When a flexor muscle contracts, the respective extensor muscle should be able to elongate freely. This is as true for the movement of individual limbs as it is for entire sections of the body. Otherwise your body will have to shorten unnecessarily and the core of your organism as well as your joints will be compressed.

5. Each movement should require the smallest possible amount of energy. In order to achieve this goal, movement impulses must not be obstructed anywhere. They should rather be able to reverberate throughout the entire structure so that the whole body participates in the movement. This will make it

more flowing and graceful. Furthermore, upper body segments must be well supported from below. (Fig. 4, p.18)

6. Approximating symmetry of left and right body-halves: This may include a certain amount of asymmetry since the left and the right side of the body are not the same inside: Most organs are not paired. Moreover, individual factors, such as left- or right-handedness, stand in the way of perfect symmetry.

7. The paired joints of left and right body-halves should be on a horizontal. If you draw lines through left and right ankle, knee, hip joint, wrist, elbow and shoulder, they should be in a horizontal plane parallel to the ground.

8. Freeing the breath will be achieved by creating enough inside space and sufficient mobility for the breathing structures to expand well.

9. Increasing sensitivity for the workings and sensations of your body as well as increasing awareness/mindfulness of what happens around you will open the spatial, emotional and interpersonal context for more harmonious movement.

Bear in mind that all these objectives are interrelated and that working on any one of them will help the others.

c. How We Go About Achieving The Goals of Rolfing

Generally speaking, we want to restore proper tension of the myofasciae, allow them to occupy enough space and have their layers and parts relate to each other well. This requires two things: differentiation and integration.

Differentiation is the functional separation of body-parts and layers, which allows them to move freely and independently of each other. Integration, on the other hand, enables all the body-parts to cooperate and constitute a more complex entity on a higher level of organization. This will make the body move more efficiently and gracefully. Both aspects - differentiation and integration - are present in each Rolfing session.

One way to achieve differentiation is by loosening and opening up adhesions. In a not so well-differentiated body, neighboring muscles are often "glued" together so that when we move, we have to engage muscles that are neither meant nor necessary for that particular movement. During a Rolfing session, the Rolfer releases these adhesions while the client performs very specific movements. This will help him/her gain awareness and integrate a better movement pattern. It will also teach the nervous system that a specific movement is possible in a simpler, more effective way. In this way, the hands-on work and the educational aspects of Rolfing complement each other to allow muscles to reclaim their appropriate space and proper functioning.

Differentiation also includes stretching chronically shortened fascia and muscles. However, the way we do it in Rolfing, stretching is not a purely mechanical event. It, too, involves a learning process in the nervous system. Muscles and even more so their fascial envelopes have stretch receptors. They react to a slow but substantial stretching of the tissue by telling the central nervous system to permanently lengthen the fibers of the tissue. Therefore, manual stretching by the Rolfer in combination with the client's active movement participation allows the body make lasting changes in the tensional relationships within its myofascial system.

The aspect of integration is most clearly present when your Rolfer considers the internal connections and interrelations that are typical of your particular body-structure. He/she will do that anew in every single Rolfing session. The work that is done in one area of the body not only changes that body-part, but also influences the way that part functions within the larger context of the whole organism. Therefore, by working one area, your Rolfer may intend to achieve major effects in a completely different place. As it is so complex, integrating a structure is the far more difficult aspect of Rolfing. To achieve true integration, it is essential to find a structural balance that caters to the various possibilities and needs of each individual client.

When we try to explain Rolfing, we could also describe it as a predominantly nonverbal form of communication between Rolfer and client. This communication develops on several different, yet connected levels and induces long-term change in the structure. One such level is neuromotor sensation. Rolfing provides enhanced neuromotor feedback for your brain about what happens in your muscles and fasciae as you move. This feedback will help your nervous system give up old, ingrained movement habits and develop new possibilities, better ways to move, instead. It can also help rediscover lost possibilities, of course. The connective tissue will be induced to continue reorganizing its spatial web after the series of Rolfing sessions has been completed.

The second level of nonverbal communication has to do with somatic awareness. Rolfing will help you become better aware of the wealth of sensations in your body. Feeling more, and more clearly, will support you in being more careful of the positive and negative influences your world may have on your body and soul. Moreover, the Rolfing process will further a growing sense of the inner vertical line and the wonderful complexity of your organism. It can help you develop an intuitive "feel" for situations and an understanding of how you react and relate to your surroundings by adopting specific postures and movements.

The third level of nonverbal communication concerns the emotional realm. During a Rolfing session or in between Rolfing sessions, emotional releases may happen. People may laugh, cry, become angry or feel relieved. Moreover, physical as well as emotional trauma, which can be stored in tissues and in the autonomic nervous system, may surface with Rolfing. This can happen in the form of unconscious somatic reactions, as conscious memory or new understanding. Your Rolfer will provide the space and support for you to deal with such feelings and reactions.

Rolfers do not normally provide talk-therapy like most psychotherapies, although in certain circumstances talking may of course be helpful. Instead, Rolfers predominantly work on the level of the autonomic nervous system (ANS). When physical or emotional trauma is adressed in a Rolfing session, the ANS - simply speaking - starts a process of nervous system charge, in which the sympathetic branch is dominant, followed by a period of discharge, in which the parasympathetic branch takes over.

Allowing this cycle to happen, and, most importantly, to complete, requires sensitive and skillful support, which your Rolfer can provide. In this way, Rolfing can initiate spontaneous self-healing processes, which promote a lasting, adaptable balance for the ANS. Good balance in the ANS will promote psychological equilibrium.

Rolfers have a wide array of techniques available to attain the goals of Rolfing Structural Integration. The most prominent are of course myofascial techniques. Other techniques, such as craniosacral or visceral manipulation, have been taken from the osteopathic tradition. Various methods to develop sensory awareness and specific movement education are also included.

What happens in the Rolfing process?

Usually, the Rolfing process takes the form of a basic series of 10 sessions, with each session lasting about 60-90 minutes. In this basic series, the entire body will be worked in a wholistic way. In chapter 3, I am going to illustrate the build-up and approach of the basic series in more detail, so here is only a general guidline: Rolfing proceeds from superficial to deeper layers of tissue. After all the layers have been addressed, we balance the deep with the superficial parts of the structure. Another thread of this process is to mainly restructure from the base of the feet upwards.

Each of the ten sessions has specific themes with certain structural and functional goals. However, what looks like an almost rigidly systematic approach actually provides the basis for very creative work, which enables the Rolfer to precisely address the particular needs of each client. In this way, the frame of the series is able to encompass a wide variety of actual work, so that each session may look very different with different clients.

For example, while one individual may tend to hold himself rigidly upright and therefore lacks moblity, the other may be in a slouching position and have hyper-mobile joints. While one client may have high arches and a forward tilted pelvis, the next may have collapsed arches and a backward tilted pelvis. Some people may need greater stability and better grounding, while others will benefit from an increase in flexibility and lightness. Furthermore, structural problems may turn out to be of secondary importance in a session if psychological issues surface. Chronic back pain can be an issue for Rolfing, but so can increasing the range of a dancer's expression.

Rolfing is about finding the best possible development, whatever that may be for a particular person, problem or situation in life. That's why the Rolfing process is both systematic as well as personal and tailored to the needs of each individual client.

An initial interview provides you (and your Rolfer) with the opportunity to clarify your needs and expecta-tions. You will most likely discuss the overall state of your health and be asked about illnesses or injuries. General information about your life may also be relevant. Many Rolfers will take pictures of your body from the front, back and sides before the first session and after you have completed the series. This will allow you to see how you have changed. It will also help your Rolfer prepare for the sessions.

A Certified Rolfer is trained to "read" body-structures and movement patterns, to see changes and improvement. What is just as important for the Rolfing process, however, is the client's capability to become aware of the changes that are being initiated by Rolfing, and his/her willingness to welcome them and use the new possibilities.

That is not as easy as it sounds. Of course, if you come to Rolfing you have some willingness to change. But we all harbor two sides: a desire for change when there is a problem as well as a reluctance to give up what is used and familiar. After all, your structure is your very own, you are used to it, and it has done you good service, at least for a while. Otherwise you would not have developed it the way you have. To replace your individual pattern with something new and at first unfamiliar can be quite challenging. It means embarking on the unknown. Feelings of uncertainty or unease can be part of that process, especially if your body-structure has developed largely in response to emotions; it has manifested in flesh your individual way of feeling and expressing yourself, the way you respond to the world.

Another factor may impede our willingness and capacity for change: believing that, in actual reality, we *cannot* change all that much. This may sound paradoxical. But consider how often you have experienced a situation in life when all efforts were futile. You were either not able or not allowed to do as you wanted. Have you never heard your parents or your doctor say, "There is no way to change this condition, you will just have to accept it."? Have you never heard: "That runs in the family, can't help it."? Moreover, the assumption that a certain body structure will largely remain the same throughout their lives, is still widespread.

Sometimes making the experience that you can, in fact, change is an essential part of the Rolfing process. Your new structure will allow more choices, which may at times create anxiety and you will definitely have to take over responsibility for yourself. However, you will also gain a lot of freedom and feel much better. Of course sometimes it may also be relevant to perceive and accept consciously limitations that have developed in the course of a lifetime and learn to be creative in dealing with them.

What do I need to contribute if I want to be rolfed?

If you want to be rolfed, you should be prepared to look at your physical as well as mental limitations. You should be willing to take over responsibility for yourself and for your personal growth, and intend to use your new-found potential after the series has been completed.

You should be ready to honestly explore when and how you are stressing yourself enough to bring on physical symptoms. Finally, you should be prepared to cooperate with your Rolfer rather than expect to be passive as he/she does the work. Rolfing can only catalyze self-regulation and self-healing. Of course, it is absolutely legitimate and reasonable to expect significant help. However, a Rolfer is not a type of "surgeon", who will eliminate old behavioral patterns from your body and implant new ones.

The fact that Rolfing works like a catalyst contains a positive aspect: balance with gravity is already blue-printed by nature in each living organism. Therefore we "only" need to create space for the organism to unfold. Actually, this is one reason why Rolfing tends to produce substantial and long-lasting results within a comparatively short amount of time.

What happens after the Basic 10 Series?

Naturally, in some cases the basic ten sessions will not be enough. Therefore, it is possible to take more Rolfing sessions after a consolidation period of usually about half a year. Observing such a break is advantageous because the results of the first ten sessions will continue to effect and change your structural and movement patterns for a while. It is a good idea to give yourself time to complete that process. Afterwards, post-ten sessions can be taken to tackle as yet unresolved issues or to refresh the work that has been done. Furthermore, advanced sessions provide the opportunity to further improve and build upon what you have already achieved.

Moreover, you can continue to work on the quality of your movement patterns by taking special movement sesssions with a Rolf Movement Practicioner.

It is possible to take Rolfing sessions to assist psychotherapy. Releasing psychological blocks with a somatic method like Rolfing can certainly support the psycho-theraeutic process. Conversely, psychological issues problems that surface in the Rolfing process may sometimes require additional attention of a psychotherapist.

How permanent are the results of Rolfing?

All living organisms strive for a higher level of organization and try to evolve a more refined complexity of their patterns. Add to that the fact that gravity reinforces indirectly body structures which are well-adapted to it and you have already two elements that will support permanency. Moreover, the balanced movement patterns that are developed in the Rolfing process will enhance balance in the body structure.

In addition, by the ensemble acting of tissues and nervous system, the organism will regain its capacity to self-regulate and release tension. For example, you may experience a bout of hypertension in the neck and shoulder area and find after a couple of days that it has disappeared "all by itself". Before your Rolfing these tensions probably have been chronic ones.

Experience shows that people who have been rolfed are better able to cope with physical as well as with emotionional stress. However, the old saying "Use it or lose it" applies. You will need to put your newfound sensitivity into action by honoring your body's signals when mus-

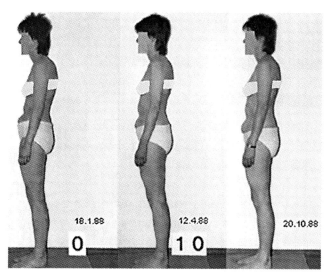

Fig. 5 Young woman before Rolfing, after Rolfing and half a year later

cular tension or pain remind you to be more considerate and caring with yourself.

Of course, life may confront anyone with a situation that throws them somewhat off balance again, such as severe illness, an accident, a job that is physically demanding or repetitive, or a psychological crisis. Post-ten Rolfing sessions can help cope and bring the system back to a harmonious balance.

How painful is Rolfing?

Rolfing is different for everyone. Some people feel only a welcome release in tension; others may experience quite intense sensations in some parts of their bodies as chronically tight tissues are starting to "melt". This can be described as a kind of pain, but it is mostly clearly linked with a sensation of relief and well-being.

Clinical pain research has shown that the sensation of pain is not a *direct* reaction to a sensory stimulus. Rather, any stimulus is transmitted across a large number of intermittent receptors and "interpretors" in nerves and the brain before we register pain, or any other sensation, for that part. In this way, stimuli are filtered and given significance by the peripheral and central nervous system. Life experiences play a big part in this process. Someone who has experienced a lot of pain in his/her life, may be predisposed toward that particular sensation and thus respond more quickly and strongly to intense stimuli.

Another person may have had to repress painful emotions such as sadness or despair repeatedly. When that happens, the emotions do not just go away. Instead, they are stored in the autonomic nervous system or held by chronic tension in parts of the body. In Rolfing, such repressed emotions may surface in the form of physical pain. Of course, the body may also store memories of injuries or surgical interventions in tissues. Unconscious fear of change may also be transformed into painful sensations. So, the pain is usually not produced by Rolfing. Rolfing only assists in bringing old pains to the surface sometimes so that they can be addressed and ultimately resolved.

Remember, though: Whenever disturbing or painful sensations you may feel are approaching your personal limit at this particular moment, you can (and should) let your Rolfer know by simply saying "Stop".

Choosing a Practitioner

One of the most important factors in any therapeutic or learning process is a relation of mutual trust between client and therapist/teacher. That is of course true for Rolfing, too. The initial interview and the first session provide a good opportunity for both Practitioner and client to find out if they feel confident that they can productively work with each other. A client should always ask him/herself: Do I feel that I can entrust myself to this person?

One aspect to determine trust is always the qualification of the practitioner. Only people who have been trained by the *Rolf Institute for Structural Integration* are entitled to use the registered servicemark *Rolfing*®. However, there are some other schools of Structural Integration that are truly related and somewhat similar to Rolfing. The best-known are the *Guild for Structural Integration* and *Hellerwork*.

Another aspect of choosing a practitioner is of course the fact that every Rolfer will have a slightly different focus, bringing his/her personal background and experience to the work.

2. Where Can Rolfing Help?

People who come to Rolfing are generally motivated by one of the following three conditions:

a) They feel limited in their range of motion or seem to be forever struggling with bad posture. This may be linked with chronic pain.

b) They use the medium of physical expression in their professional or private lives and would like to expand their possibilities. This includes many athletes, dancers, actors, singers and people who practise Yoga, Aikido or the like.

c) They want to work with their bodies in order to be able to deal with psychological issues better or to realize their full human potential.

In actual reality, these motives are rarely as clear-cut. Most people come with any combination of the three. However, I will treat them separately in order to be able to describe each theme more clearly.

a. Limited Range of Motion and Postural Problems

First an important disclaimer: Rolfing is not a medical procedure that relieves symptoms. A Rolfer does not diagnose or treat sickness. Therefore, Rolfing can not replace medical attention. If necessary, we will ask a client to see a doctor. If you expect Rolfing to alleviate physical symptoms, you should be aware that any relief you may get will "only" be a side-effect of improving your body-structure.

Still, Rolfing can be beneficial for both sick as well as healthy people. Naturally, symptoms that are caused by structural imbalances can improve when you receive Rolfing work. However, Rolfing does not concentrate on problem-areas but employs a wholistic perception in looking at the entire organism. In consistency with that, Rolfing seeks to restructure the body gradually which will allow the client to learn to cope with local issues, for example damaged discs, more effectively. Many issues such as lower back pain can become obsolete in this process.

Some medical conditions, however, are mostly a contraindication to Rolfing and allow at best very limited work. These include cancer, severe heart diseases, multiple sclerosis, severe (!) spastic disorders, advanced osteoporosis, brain damage, psychosis. The initial interview will clarify whether you can be Rolfed. If there are any doubts, your doctor will be asked to decide.

Let us now have a look at some body-oriented issues that can be tackled with Rolfing.

Spinal problems

Ideally, your spine should have a slight, flexible S-curvature, which allows the weight of your body to be evenly transmitted down and the impact of small shocks to be well absorbed. Unfortunately, the ideal S-shape is very often compromised.

For example, the curvatures of the cervical spine and the low back (lordoses) as well as the complimentary curvatures of the mid-back and sacrum (kyphoses) may be too strong. You can see this in people with a "sway-back". It is very often coupled with a too far forward-downward tilted pelvis. In this scenario, the cervical and lumbar portions of the spine will be in front of the vertical centerline, locked into their curvature and held by chronically shortened muscles in the back. Being *in front* of the plumbline, the weight of the chest and the head will lack support from underneath, which explains why the muscles of the mid-back and at the transition of the thoracic to the lumbar spine are so often tense and aching.

However, releasing the tension in the back is not enough to alleviate this problem. The position of the pelvis must be addressed also: If it is tilted forward and down, the sacrum will also be tilted forward and down and it will take the lumbar vertebrae along. So, as long as the pelvis has not found a more horizontal position, the back-problems will not significantly improve.

If the S-curvature of the spine is too straight, on the other hand, the spine loses part of its resilience. In that case, trouble usually occurs at the transition from the lumbar spine to the sacrum. Very often, the fifth lumbar vertebra will have slipped forward while pelvis and sacrum are tilted backwards. Disc problems are a common result.

These or any other "weak spots" in the spine will deteriorate more easily. In order to fulfill its function well, the spine needs to be permeable for vibration to freely transmit stress, strains and movement impulses just like the rest of the body.

Let's have a look at what happens when you walk: With every step that hits the ground, a shockwave is sent upwards into the body. If the structure is free and resilient, the energy of this wave can reverberate through the whole body and be well-absorbed. (The fibula is designed as a shock-absorber for walking but it performs this function well only when it "floats" in the surrounding tissues freely.)

If, on the other hand, some joints in the body are hypermobile while others are too inflexible to allow easy transmission of the movement impulses, the hypermobile joints, which are less stable anyway, will receive too great a strain. For instance, when the thoracic spine is rigid and fixed while the fifth lumbar and sacrum instable, each step will send a shockwave into this hypermobile low back area. Painful degenerative processes are the result.

Degenerating discs can get relief if we manage to reestablish movement in the unflexible, immobile parts of the body. Furthermore, changing the structure of legs and pelvis helps if they can provide a better supportive basis for the spine

Whether Rolfing can ameliorate chronic disc problems will depend on the degree of degeneration: Is the fibrous outer ring of the disc still somewhat elastic? How much damage has already happened in the nervous tissue? If the nerves are damaged, the area will remain painful even after the structural strain has been taken off the nerve until the nervous tissue has regenerated. In these cases acupuncture or other additional remedies can be very helpful.

Your Rolfer will, in any case, work with such problem areas in a very careful and gentle way and explore more indirect ways of influencing the area: It is essential to help the body let go of those postural adaptations to the pain which have developed in acute phases. These compensatory postures are meant to keep strain from the painful area. However, they inhibit movement and consequently tend to ingrain the problem into the structure.

Did you know that almost everybody has a scoliosis? A scoliosis is constituted by two or more sidebends in the spine and the resulting rotations and counterrotations of vertebrae around the vertical axis. Being born creates a slight scoliosis in everyone. If it remains slight, there will not be any problems. You will probably never even notice your birth-scoliosis. However, if other factors reinforce the bends, the scoliosis can become abnormal. The line between normal and abnormal scoliosis is, as in other structural "abnormities", not a sharp one. One of the factors that can worsen a scoliosis, for example, becomes present when a child is forced to grow up too fast - in a physical (child labor) or in an emotional sense. When the bones grow faster than the musculature, the spine will react with sidebending and rotating. Other factors that can worsen a scoliosis are legs of differing length or the aging process.

An essential part of Rolfing a scoliosis is to lengthen chronically short tissues to allow the spine to lift up. Lengthening the spine in this way can reduce the rotations of individual vertebrae and diminish the sidebends. Scolioses of course require special pattern-specific work from the Rolfer. Relations between the spine and the rest of the body need particular attention. Moreover,

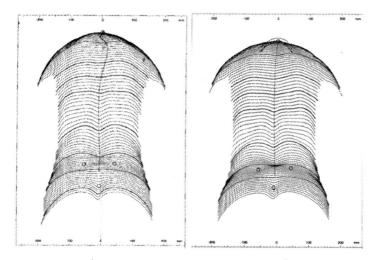

Fig. 6 Photometric 3D-Reconstruction of a spine
before and after ten Rolfing sessions

connective tissue restrictions in the visceral (organ)
space of the torso are sometimes causes for an abnormal
scoliosis and need to be addressed. Rolfing can usually
not make a scoliosis disappear alltogether, but a decrease
in severity is often possible (Fig. 6).

I have already mentioned low back pain in the discus-
sion of spinal problems above, and pointed out the fact
that the positions of pelvis and sacrum play a vital part.
A forward tilted sacrum may, moreover, result in low
back pains in the time of female menstruation because
the uterus and the sacrum are connected by ligaments.

This problem can be aggravated when the pelvic floor muscles are shortened or hypertense.

The same structural relations can explain why women often experience back pain in pregnancy: The added weight of the fetus may pull the base of the sacrum forward and down more, so that the low and mid back have to compensate with increasing tension resulting in pain. Rolfing can help bring the weight closer to the plumbline, that is, back into and over the pelvis. Support from underneath can be improved by aligning the legs under the body better. The back itself will of course also need some work.

However, Rolfing is not advisable in all stages of the pregnancy and generally has to be gentler. Very often, though, giving birth is much easier if a woman has taken Rolfing sessions before becoming pregnant because her pelvis will be more flexible. Furthermore, her pelvic floor and the surrounding ligaments will stretch more easily.

The base of the sacrum can not only be tilted too far forward or back, it can also be tipped to one side. If that is the case, the iliosacral joint between hip-bone and sacrum will often be unstable on one side and inflexible on the other.

Problems in legs and feet

The changes happening in a body structure during Rolfing often start a maturation process that may have come to a standstill in childhood or puberty. For example, flat feet do not have to be collapsed arches. They can be the feet of a child that never matured enough to develop arches. After all, flat feet are perfectly normal in an infant before he/she starts walking. A lot of feet actually get stuck in that phase. Rolfing may be able to restart the development process. However, the results will initally be felt rather than seen, since developing a visibly stronger arch takes some time.

Structural problems in the legs often show in rotations of the thighs. Inward rotated thighs will usually result in O-legs, whereas turned out thighs will produce X-legs. If the rotations and consequent malfunctions persist over many years, the bones of thigh and leg will adapt and change their shape, too. The shape of the bones of course limits corrections that are possible with Rolfing. However, functional improvements can be expected so that walking will become more secure. This will have positive effects on the joints, too. In the long run, moving in a structurally more balanced way may even induce the bones to somewhat normalize their shape. Obviously, this is a long-term project.

In many people, the joints of hip, knee and ankle are not well aligned. For instance, the femurs may be rotated inwards while the lower legs and feet are turned out. In that case, the joint-axes of the knees are pointing across while the joint-axes of the ankles are directed away from each other. This configuration will tremendously strain the knees when you are walking. With each step, the knee will start to move forwards and towards the other leg following the direction of its structural axis. As you want to walk straight forward, though, the cross-impulse has to be corrected to the outside in the latter part of the step. Therefore, the normal hinge-like movement of walking is replaced with a kind of swerving motion for which the knee is not designed. Moreover, all of this will put your weight more on the ouside edges of the foot, which increases the risk of twisting your ankle.

If one of the three joints of the leg is unstable and hypermobile, the reason is usually that at least one of the others is too inflexible. An equally common correlation appears when one hip-joint is too inflexible, so that the other has to compensate the motion and becomes unstable.

Differences in leg-length can be adjusted as long as they do not stem from an actual difference in the length of the bones. Causes of differing leg-length which can be successfully addressed are, for example, a collapsed arch or a compressed hip-joint in the shorter leg.

Chronic joint arthrosis

Arthrosis of a joint describes a disturbance of normal tissue-metabolism which results in degenerative processes in the tissues of and around the joint. Overproduction of collagen fibers and calcium deposits tends to decrease range of motion. What you eat is certainly often decisive for joint metabolism.

However, what looks like a genuine arthrosis may actually be a pseudo-arthrosis: arthritc degeneration and pain in a joint can also originate from shortened, malpositioned ligaments and muscles. In that case the metabolism of the joints gets disrupted because the tissues are too bunched up to be pervious. The joint may be so compressed that adequate metabolism is simply squeezed off.

Scientific studies have shown a correlation between arthrosis of the hip-joint and a forward-downward tilted pelvis. In such cases, improving joint-mechanics as well as the perviousness of the surrounding tissues so that fluid exchanges can happen across body-segments, can significantly improve the person's subjective condition as well as her range of motion. Of course this does not make medical treatment of other contributing factors unnecessary. If your are having an acute inflammatory condition of the joint, you should not be rolfed in that area.

Some medical terms are not very clearly defined. Among them are "rheumatism" or "Morbus Bechterew". Generaly speaking, Bechterew's disease describes a process of bending and rigidification of the spine, which usually starts in the lumbar area. In the intermission periods between acute inflammatory phases, the person suffering from Bechterew reacts favorably to Rolfing if the disease is not yet in its advanced stages. If the Bechterew-patient is willing to consider regular Rolfing sessions over a longer period of time, an increase in mobility and some regaining of upright stance may be possible. Even though expectations should not be too high, stopping or at least slowing down the ossification process can mean a significant improvement. It can, however, only be attained when Rolfing is included in an overall regime of diet, lots of movement and possibly psychotherapy.

Many people suffer from inflexibility. However, a considerable number of people have to deal with hypermobile joints. If the problem is too much mobility, Rolfing will focus more on stabilization and integration than of loosening and differentiattion.

Shoulder and neck problems

Shoulder and neck problems can be the result of so many different, complex sets of circumstances that the scope of this book does not allow me to discuss them all. We can safely state, though, that chronic tension in the shoulder and neck area is directly or indirectly a product of the overall body-structure. That is why massages that are limited to the area of the tension (i.e. shoulder and neck) will not produce satisfying results in the long run.

Often, the source of the trouble is a lack of support from the lower body-parts. If they are not properly supported from underneath, the muscles of shoulder and neck bear sole responsibility for holding the head upright. This is asking too much of them. For example: if the chest is collapsed in front, it will pull the shoulders and neck with it and out of vertical alignment. The shoulder-girdle and the head come to rest *in front* of the plumbline, so that shoulder and neck muscles in the back are forced to tense up and shorten in their attempt to keep the head up. The collapsed chest, in turn, may be held down by shortened abdominal muscles.

Chronic headaches and migraines

Headaches, too, are often a result of structural imbalances. If, for example, the joint between the skull and the first cervical vertebra gets jammed because of shortened muscle and conntective tissue, the vertebral artery can be compressed and the flow of blood congested. As a consequence, blood will build up ahead of the constriction and may squeeze the suboccipital nerve. This in turn will increase the constriction and may actually start a vicious cycle of frequent headaches.

Another factor that can impede circulation in the vertebral artery is too much of a curve in the cervial spine. Even minute vertebral displacements there will disturb circulation because the vertebral artery is threaded through small holes in the transverse processes of the vertebrae.

Headaches can also be a long-term result of accidents (whiplash syndrome). If structural misalignments in the area of head, neck, shoulders and spine are not corrected after the injured ligaments, blood vessels and muscles have healed, they can manifest in various symptoms much later.

TMJ and problems with the muscles of mastication

One of the key areas for hypertension encompasses the joints of the jaw and the muscles of mastication. If the muscles of mastication are chronically tense, people may be grinding their teeth while they sleep and develop muscular pains. These symptoms will often travel to the neck and head areas and produce tension and headaches. Moreover, bruxism - that is what nightly teeth-grinding is called in dental care - will wear off the tooth substance prematurely and can lead to bite-anomalies.

The Rolfing approach to this, just like to any other hypertension problem, is of course not limited to releasing the afflicted musculature. We have to take into account a host of other factors like, for example, the relation between jaw, skull and cervical spine. Also, movement patterns and tone in the tissues surrounding the joints may differ considerably from left to right side. Furthermore, long periods of tension and/or painful cramps in the muscles of mastication generate a state of high charge in the autonomic nervous system, which tends to increase muscular tension even more. This vicious cycle can only be reversed gradually.

Developmental issues and the aging process

Development and aging are often themes of Rolfing. Basically, Rolfing can be a benefit to people of all ages. When we work with children, we naturally focus more on their current development than on their life-story. Moreover, we have to take into account the characteristic structural aspects of each developmental stage as well. In addition, we will adapt the work to a child's capabilities and needs, working more playfully and in shorter sessions than with adults. Obviously, structural imbalances will impede development less if they are addressed as early as possible.

When working with the elderly, we also have to take developmental principles into account. Typical physical aspects of aging include: an increase of fibrosis or calcifications in the soft tissues, more deposits of metabolic waste or a diminishing range of motion. Rolfing often succeeds in slowing down such aspects of the aging process, in lessening their impact or sometimes even reversing them.

The issues that can be addressed with Rolfing and the underlying angle of view which I have discussed in this chapter are far from exhaustive. However, I have tried to provide a general idea of how Structural Integration can benefit the entire human organism.

b. Improving and Refining Somatic Expression and Movement

Even though you might not be free from the type of ailment I have described above, you may be interested mainly in increasing your somatic awareness and developing your fine motor skills. Rolfing is great for that because it is more than a mere tool to work on health problems.

Many Rolfing clients use their bodies as a physical medium in their professional lives. They come to Rolfing to increase their possibilities. For example, a professional

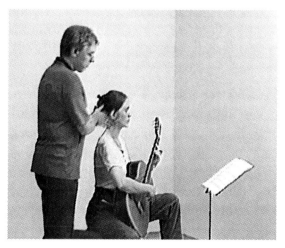

Fig. 7 Rolf Movement education
for a professional musician

dancer may have great flexibility in her legs and hip joints, yet be dissatisfied with her range of expression in the shoulder and chest area. Another artist may need to put his/her body into a highly specific posture to practise or perform, which can interfere with artistic expression. The typical posture of professional violinists, for instance, often produces chronic hypertension of the neck and shoulders and a structural twist of the torso to the left side. This not only feels uncomfortable at times, it may also interfere with the free flow of musical expression and the fine qualities of the sound. Rolfing can provide a means to resolve problems that have already developed. It can also assist in finding a way to perform so that the postural hazards of the profession are avoided.

A large number of (professional) dancers gained some profit from Rolfing. For example, the British dancer and choreograph *Russell Maliphant*, who eventually became a Rolfer himself.

People who are involved in sports often report that Rolfing has improved their mobility and coordination. No matter if you are a student who likes skiing, a businessperson who regularly plays tennis or a physician practicing belly-dance, your movement will become more effortless, effective and graceful, as your body gains greater structural balance and smoother muscle activity.

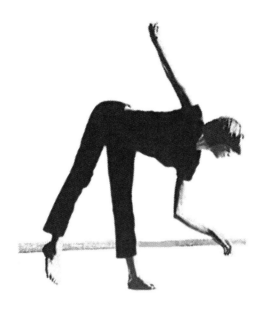

Fig. 8 Moving through lengthening
the body instead of shortening
can help dancers to prevent injuries

Jose Augusto Menegatti, former coach of the Brazilian National Volleyball Team, was rolfed and later trained as a Rolfer himself. When he was asked how Rolfing could improve the performance of a volleyball player, he explained:

> "Most of the practice time of the players is usually spent developing specific parts of their bodies - stronger arms, faster legs, etc. Rolfing, on the

other hand, allows the players to feel their bodies as an integrated whole. The kind of physical awareness they gain from Rolfing enables them to use their strength in a better balanced way, to move more freely and to play more effectively.

Moreover, Rolfing allows the athletes to breathe better which diminishes fatigue and shortens their recovery-times. Also, breathing patterns change with stress. Athletes who have been rolfed are better aware of their breathing and thus better able to relax and control their stress level.

But the most important aspect for the game is that Rolfing opens up spaces in the body, which allows the players to move in a well-integrated way. And I am not talking about the physical only. I am talking about the entire person. The higher level of integration in each member of the team furthers respect for his teammates and promotes the team spirit. The players get to feel that cooperating is good. Individual players do not try to show off as stars any more, which most likely would cost the team points."

Menegatti admits, though, that "not everybody is ready for Rolfing. Rolfing stimulates change and personal growth. And not everyone is willing to allow that."

A scientific study which was conducted in California in 1973 corroborates Menegatti's observations. It demonstrated that the muscles of rolfed individuals contract for a shorter period of time than those of unrolfed people when doing the same movements. Thus, energy expenditure becomes more even. Moreover, muscle activity in those areas of the body that are not directly involved in the movement decreases so that less energy is wasted on unnecessary muscle activity. In general, movements tend to be more fluid, more spacious and less forced.

People who practise yoga often report that their sensations when doing the yoga positions are deeper than before Rolfing. They are better able to synchronize the motions and relax while holding the positions.

A psychotherapist who I worked with described another form of increased body-awareness. With Rolfing, she learned to refine her body awareness and to respect her own physical sensations more. As a result, she was better aware of her clients' physical being. This opened up another way for her to learn about her clients' personalities and emotional problems.

Lots of people make this kind of experience in various contexts after their own Rolfing process. They become more appreciative of the ways their fellow-humans are special physically as well as mentally when they have developed their own sensory awareness.

c. Finding Emotional Balance and Developing Human Potential

Rolfing is not a form of psychotherapy. However, many people perceive changes during the Rolfing process that are similar to what they might experience in psychotherapy. Let me show you a few examples.

Anna's story demonstrates to what extent physical and emotional tensions can be related. She was fifty years old, married, and had three sons. In the initial interview, she said that she was aware that her feelings and emotions were linked to the way she experienced her body. She suffered from severe depression, insomnia, apathy and did not like her husband. She sensed her body as extremely rigid, hard and "surrounded by a three foot thick wall".

In her first Rolfing session, she realized that she could be with herself completely, which was a new and wonderful experience. Moreover, my mindfulness made her aware of how much she missed affection in her life. She cried, releasing some emotions; that started to soft-en the almost paralyzed, depressed state she was normal-ly in.

In the following weeks she was able to sleep more and better. As we progressed through her Rolfing series, she learned to recognize her own needs more clearly. She also became aware of them sooner in her interactions with her husband and sons than before. Anna started to stand up for her needs and managed to contact the angry feelings in herself. She experienced mood swings but was happy to be able to feel the excitement of life again. These emotional changes happened parallel to the development of her body, which gained in aliveness and permeability.

Sven suffered from Bechterew's disease. In the course of his Rolfing series, he started to reflect on his illness and found that it had been providing him with a means to escape the stresses of his work. For a long time, he had not been able to acknowledge that he was feeling overwhelmed by the demands of his job. He realized, too, that he had been using his disease to get more attention from other people: His physiotherapist had been there for him for years. Becoming aware of the psychological aspects of his illness enabled Sven to let go of it somewhat. After that, Bechterew was no longer the defining factor of his life. This made greater physcial changes possible and helped him to gain more mobility and self-esteem. His obsessive-compulsive tendencies decreased and he started to enjoy life more.

Harry was still a young man but suffered from back pain and overall hypertension. He had been working extremely hard to be able to build his own business. During Rolfing, he realized that his back pain was really his body's way of telling him that he was putting too much strain on himself. Harry gradually learned that it was not necessary to force everything but that he could also relax and let some things happen by themselves. He came to be more respectful of his own needs and limitations.

Marianne told me in her introductory interview that her relationship with her father had been so bad that she grew up distrusting and fearing men. Being rolfed by a male Rolfer may have provided her with the positive, body-centered experience and safe environment she needed to recognize that she did not want to spend her life avoiding men. When Marianne finally managed to acknowledge her need for a loving relationship with a man, her fear of physical contact also diminished. Moreover, she found the strength to talk to her father and rediscovered some positive feelings for him, too.

The increased stability of the feet and legs that comes with Rolfing very often generates greater stability in a more figurative sense, too. People learn to be more trustful of their ability to stay on their own feet when things are rough. They come to feel stronger and more secure.

Some people find that Rolfing improved their sex lives, too. They began to feel greater pleasure and became better aware of their sexual needs.

Just as Rolfing can jump-start physical development that got deadlocked somewhere in the body, it can also encourage emotional maturity and growth. Sometimes, psychological aspects that are less developed get to mature and catch up with the rest of the personality. In this way, Rolfing can help overcome stagnation in personal growth processes and support people in realizing their full human potential.

During the Rolfing process, habitual patterns of sensation, thought and living tend to soften up. That allows you to try new ways of meeting the challenges of life. Also, you may suddenly find it much easier to make that long-overdue decision that you have been putting off all the time.

The better your body can organize around its inner vertical line, the easier it will be for you to find your center. When your organismic self progresses in spatial organization, your life and environment will seem clearer and more defined. Your intuitive appreciation for balance in your body will increase. So will your capability to establish, maintain and further adapt order in your life.

The scientific study I have mentioned earlier demonstrated that Rolfing causes the right brain hemisphere to be more active in solving a "right brain task". Right brain tasks include intuitive and analogous thinking, processing physical sensations and wholistic perception. The left brain hemisphere is in charge of logical and analytical thinking, math and language. Another study mentions that people who have been rolfed tend to be more accepting of themselves and more able to live in the here and now. They develop better relationship skills and are more open to their emotions.

Sometimes people come to Rolfing when their progress in psychotherapy seems to have come to a standstill. Very often, Rolfing can provide an impetus for the unconscious to resume the psychotherapeutic process. On the other hand, you may have successfully gone through an emotional crisis or changes of personality, but your body-structure has not adapted. If that is the case, Rolfing can contribute by rounding off, or completing the psychological changes on the physical level.

Physical handicaps such as bad posture, an awkward gait, or clumsiness can generate feelings of insecurity and inferiority, especially in children and teenagers. It is obvious how much getting rid of the physical handicap will contribute to their well-being and an unstunted emotional development.

When I work with people as a Rolfer, I am always responsive to their emotional and spiritual world, even if someone does not come to Rolfing with those issues in mind. As a client, you should also try to be open towards your soul even if you are mainly looking for physical change.

If, on the contrary, you are primarily interested in gaining psychological support to help you meet the challenges of life, I try to determine in the initial interview whether Rolfing is the way to go or whether psychotherapy or a combination of the two would be better. Generally speaking, if you tend to feel emotional problems strongly in your body, if emotions create chronic hypertension, Rolfing is definitely a good possibility - with or without accompanying psychotherapy.

3. The Basic-Ten-Series

In this chapter, I will outline the themes of the ten basic sessions of Rolfing. My main intention is to provide accompanying information for those readers who are currently getting rolfed. If you are among them, I suggest you only read what is going to come up next in your series so that your attention is not diverted from your experience. If you read about later topics much in advance, you may not be able to keep in touch with the changes that are going on now so well.

However, do not expect your series to be just like the following outline in every detail! The themes and objectives of your Rolfing process may deviate more or less, depending on a number of factors. For one, every Rolfer focuses on different aspects of the work. Also, your Rolfing process will be just that: *your* Rolfing process. Thus, your motive for being rolfed and your individual body-structure will be taken into account; your Rolfer will adapt the basic themes to them. Moreover, each session may develop a certain momentum of its own, which requires flexible adjustments of the strategy. Therefore, the outline I am providing here should never be regarded as a fixed blueprint.

This is especially true for the concepts in "psychological themes" that I have included in the description of each session. Since Rolfing focuses on physical structure, psychological topics are not always addressed directly but rather in the context of your personal needs. Your motivation and individual process will determine if these or other emotional aspects play a part at all.

a. General Suggestions

Writing a diary can help you keep track of your process while you are taking Rolfing sessions. You may want to compare your weight, height and size before the first and after the last session.

If you are an athlete or work hard physically you should not push your limits during that time. You should always warm up thoroughly and be a little more careful with yourself.

Since Rolfing will activate your metabolism, it is a good idea to drink lots of fluids between the sessions, especially between the first three. That way, metabolic waste substances and toxins can be discarded from the organism more easily. In the hours before a session, you should only eat lightly. Try to get plenty of sleep the night before.

There are various ways to "open" the part of the body we are working on. One way you can help is by visualizing - even if you feel discomfort. For example, you can visualize a flower opening to full bloom, or you can imagine how you welcome the hand of your Rolfer like a helpful friend. Breathe into the areas that are being worked; visualize how you direct each breath you take. Whatever you try, be attentive and stay available for any thoughts, images, emotions or sensations that may come up.

Take some time after each session to allow your body and mind to really feel what is going on. A quiet walk can provide a good context for that. Feelings and body-awareness need some time to process before you plunge back into everyday life.

For a few days after each session, various feelings or moods can surface. Welcome them. Observe them, feel into them, allow them to happen; they are often part of your organism releasing old tensions.

If you have more energy and feel the urge to move, do it. Go dancing (a great way to allow your body to get to know itself), go swimming, do whatever you enjoy. On the other hand, you may feel a greater desire for sleep. Follow that also. If you have to sit for long periods of time, take short breaks to move a little.

Do not create a fixed image of what your body should be like. When people are going through the changes of Rolfing, as former postural and movement patterns are breaking up, they may feel tempted to "stand up straight". Putting yourself into a "good" position consciously, however, would only create new tensions. Instead, allow your body to be new and different. Appreciate your body's wisdom, and do experiment with the new movement possibilites and exercises your Rolfer teached you. Additional material you will find in the sections called "Between the Sessions".

Pay attention to what your body feels and does. If, for example, sometime during the day you realize that you are pulling your shoulders up and your belly in - you will become more aware of that through Rolfing - allow yourself to let go and return to a more natural relaxed position. Maybe you will find yourself in old patterns and postures sometimes. Be aware of them but be also aware that you have alternatives available, even if they feel a little strange at first. Explore the new qualities and note how you feel more natural, comfortable and at ease. For a while, you will go back and forth between old and new possibilities and the new will slowly become familiar. Other changes, however, will happen all "by themselves" without your every day consiousness.

Rolfing will make you more sensitive for what your body is trying to tell you. You might, for example, feel like straightening yourself instead of slouching, or you might start to feel tensions earlier than before. Watch yourself: Are you twisting when you take something off a shelf? If you have headaches, consider: what in your life is giving you a headache? Be creative in shaping your life and be creative with your movement. You can also ask your Rolfer for alternative suggestions.

After a few days, you may not be able to feel the changes that happened in the last session as clearly. They are still there! Your body has merely grown accustomed to the new way and already integrated it. There will be moments when you consciously feel the changes again, but these moments usually appear out of the blue. Working, taking a walk, or exercising may all provide instances when you are suddenly aware of the new ease and fluidity, a greater range of motion and an increase in energy.

Use these hints like a map, that will help you find *your* path of experience.

b. What The Ten Sessions Are About

The First Session

The first session provides the opportunity for you and your Rolfer to get to know different areas of your body and to establish a suitable rhythm for the work.

Body-Themes

One aim of the first session is to create more space between chest and pelvis as well as between chest and shoulder-girdle. Also, the chest should be brought into better alignment over the pelvis. Moreover, freedom of breathing will be increased. A further goal is to improve the mobility of the hip joints.

Generally speaking, the first session is designed to reestablish some of the natural tone and resilience of the big surface fascia. Special emphasis will be placed on the fasciae of the trunk.

Psychological Themes

The way we breathe directly influences the way we feel. Breath is an essential source of our life-energy. If you do not breathe in deeply enough, consider: Do I take what I need to live? What are the situations in which my breathing becomes shallow? How do I feel then? If I do not breathe out completely: Am I trying to hold onto things in my life? What are the situations in which I do not exhale enough? How do I feel then? What are the things I do not want to express or let go of?

Between Sessions 1 and 2

Sit down with your chest collapsed and take a few deep breaths in this position to explore the degree of freedom of your breathing. Then, roll your pelvis forward until you sit on the front of your sitbones. This will put your pelvis into a slight anterior tipped position and causes your chest to lift up without effort. Keep your shoulders relaxed when you take a few deep breaths again. How large is your breath now compared to before? Fig. 9 can help you with this exercise.

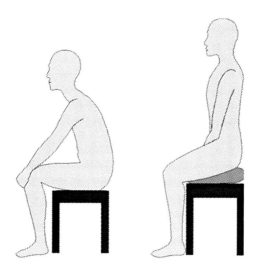

Fig. 9

The Second Session

Body-Themes

In the second session we will start to restructure the legs and the back. Proper alignment in the base of your structure (feet and legs) will improve the stability of the whole system. Moreover, the feet and legs are a key area for the transmission of movement impulses into the entire body. With each step you take, they transmit information about how smooth their mechanics are and how they meet the ground into the upper parts of the body. In addition, if your gait is well-balanced, your weight will be evenly distributed on the feet. Balanced arches and good hinging action of the ankles are important for that.

Psychological Themes

Questions to explore: Can I stand on my own feet or do I always rely on others? Am I self-supportive or dependent? Do I feel supported and secure? Do I have an opinion of my own, my own standpoint? Understanding comes from standing! Do I feel I have got firm ground under my feet or do I have my head in the clouds? Maybe my ground is too firm? Am I digging my claws into it? Do I fear change? Am I flexible enough to change my point of view now and then?

Between Sessions 2 and 3

Drink lots of fluids especially in the days following your second session; Rolfing the feet will stimulate your metabolism. If you drink enough, your body will find it easier to flush the metabolic waste substances and toxins which have accumulated over time out of your system.

A visualizing exercise which will affect your nervous system: try imagining that you have long strings attached to your kneecaps and that someone is pulling your knees horizontally forward as you walk. The two strings on your kneecaps are parallel to each other and to the ground. Alternatively, you can visualize that your knees have two headlights which shine parallel and straight forward into the direction you are walking. Do not attempt to consciously control or even "improve" the way you are walking! Just visualize either one of the images, start walking and observe. What happens? How does it feel?

The Third Session

Body-Themes

In the third session, we take a look at the sides of the body and work towards better vertical alignment. Lengthening the sides will increase front to back balance and bring the segments of the body closer to the vertical plumbline.

You can look at a number of "checkpoints" to get an idea of how balanced front and back are. These are: ears, shoulder joints, hip joints, knees and ankles. You should

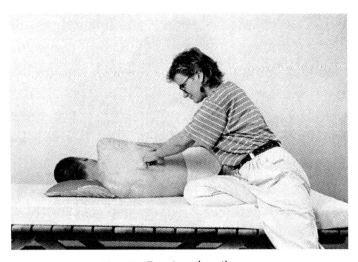

Fig. 10 Freeing the ribcage

be able to draw a vertical line trough them, with individual checkpoints being close, but not exactly on the line. In a well-balanced structure, the checkpoints of the segments will slightly deviate to the front or back. For example, at the very best the pelvis is slightly tilted forward-downward; therefore the hipjoint will come a fraction *behind* the plumbline.

Another topic of the third session is the shoulder girdle. It should be capable of unrestricted movement, and it should be resting on top of the ribcage. The arms should be relaxed, their weight hanging down from the shoulder girdle without being held. If the shoulder girdle is sufficiently unrestricted, the arms can swing freely in contralateral movement as you walk.

In the third session, we can also continue to work on breathing by expanding the space in the lumbar area and between the ribs. Especially the area around the twelfth rib has a considerable impact on the overall structure.

Psychological Themes

When I reach out with my arms, I may be doing one of two things on the symbolic-emotional level: First, to reach out is to establish (physical) contact; it can symbolize giving and receiving. Secondly, I may reach out in order to push something or somebody away; it can symbolize rejecting something, defending myself and expressing anger. Think about the double meaning of the word "arms"!

The sides of the trunk support the arms and thus symbolize support in our relations with other people – "I stand by your side". Can I ask others for help and support? Do I provide enough support for others myself? Do I hold feelings of tenderness, anger or frustration in my arms instead of expressing them? Am I sometimes unable to relax my arms because I feel insecure? Do I meet challenges in life with drooping shoulders or do I pull them back too tightly?

All or any of these themes may become relevant again in session 8 or 9.

Between Sessions 3 and 4

Now and then, sense into your shoulders and arms. Are they relaxed or are you holding them? If you feel you are tensing, imagine your arms and elbows to become heavy with the next exhalation and allow them to drop a little. Do not carry bags over one shoulder only, change sides repeatedly. When you go shopping, use two bags so that you can carry your groceries in a more balanced way.

Try breathing into your sides; fill the space between your ribs and pelvis. You can try that when you are lying down (with your knees up) as well as in standing or sitting. Feel how your sides expand as you inhale. Then try the same thing with your lower back.

The Fourth Session

Body-Themes

In sessions four to seven, we concentrate on balancing space and position of the core area of the organism. When we talk about "core", we refer to the interior space which holds the organs and viscera and is defined by surrounding muscles and fasciae. The core includes all the space from the nose and throat to the pelvic floor. Working with the core will allow the vertical inner line of the body to expand. Balancing the position of the pelvis is crucial for good core expansion and will be part of sessions 4, 5 and 6.

The aim of the fourth session is to free up and organize those tissue structures that form the boundary of the core from below. They include, of course, the pelvic floor, but also the muscles on the inside of the legs. Thus, we come back to the theme of the second session - position of feet and legs - on a deeper level. Working on the deep connective tissue sheaths close to the spine can also be part of fourth hour core-work.

Functionally, the fourth session will focus on ease and fluidity of walking as well as on the resilience of the pelvic floor. A well working pelvic floor does three things: One, it supports the intestines and the interior sexual organs. Two, it lets the breath expand downwards, and three, it allows free motion of the legs and pelvis.

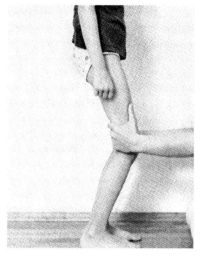

Fig. 11 Establishing a hinge
function of the joints of the legs

Psychological Themes

Psychologically, session four is about controlling and letting go. As a toddler, you were expected to learn self-control and stop wetting your diapers. Toilet-training is usually one of the first occasions where we are supposed to control ourself. It requires control of your pelvic floor muscles. Later on, self-control may have been associated with not hanging loose, not showing any feelings, or never giving up. Of course, self-control is very necessary and adequate in some situations. It makes acts of will-power and endurance possible. However, both skills - self-control as well as letting go - are important in life: in forming and maintaining relationships, for sex, at work. Fear often disturbes the delicate balance between controlling and letting go. Do I let fear interfere with this balance in my life? What are situations which make me contract my pelvic floor? Do I have control over my pelvic floor muscles at all?

Between Sessions 4 and 5

Try contracting and relaxing your pelvic floor when you walk. How does either action affect your gait? If you have difficulty contracting (such a lack of tone in the pelvic floor muscles is more common in women), exercise the muscles: Imagine that you want to interrupt the flow of urine and contract the muscles you need to do that. (However, avoid to contract your belly and butt!) Relax, and repeat a couple of times. Try breathing gently into the pelvic floor area from time to time. Direct your breath. You can do that in standing, sitting or lying on your back, with your knees up.

The Fifth Session

Body-Themes

In session five, we continue working on the core by re-balancing the pelvic floor with the respiratory diaphragm, and the deep layers of the low back with the front sheaths of the torso. This includes establishing a tensional balance between deep and superficial abdominal musculature. (Fig. 12)

One of the key structures of the body, which are espe-

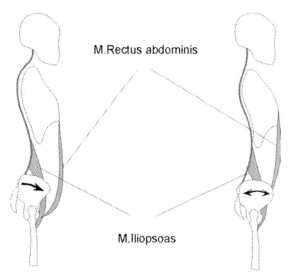

M.Rectus abdominis

M.Iliopsoas

Fig. 12

cially important in the context of the fifth session, are the two iliopsoas muscles. Actually, each iliopsoas in turn comprises two muscles. They have one name because they share a common tendon. If the muscles of the iliopsoas have adequate tone and resilience, the lumbar spine can organize itself properly. Moreover, a functioning iliopsoas will allow torso, pelvis and legs to acquire a balanced position relative to each other (compare the right drawing in Fig. 12). The left picture shows clearly what can happen if length and tone of iliopsoas and long abdominal muscle (rectus abdominis) are out of balance: The pelvis will tilt forward and down, the belly will drop forward and the low back will arch into a swayback.

We resolve deep restrictions within abdomen and chest by working on the fascial envelopes and ligaments of the organs. Organ adhesions and restrictions often cause structural problems from deep inside the body.

One of the funcional goals of session five concerns gait. There are basically two types of walking: the extrinsic and the intrinsic mode. In extrinsic walking, the thigh and leg are lifted forward by extrinsic, more superficial muscles (mostly the rectus femuris muscle shown in Fig. 13). This way of walking is very common. In intrinsic walking, on the other hand, the movement impulse starts with the action of the deep psoas muscle (the right picture in Fig. 13). The intrinsic walk is effortless and much more graceful, but it is only possible when the psoas muscle is resilient and well balanced with the extrinsic long thigh muscles.

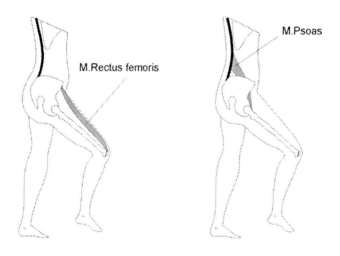

Fig. 13

Other functional goals of session five include uninhibited breathing into belly and chest as well as adequate space and mobility of the organs. If the organs are free from spatial and movement restrictions, they will function better. Moreover, structural balance of the inside and outside of the trunk will increase.

Psychological Themes

Belly and chest are often used as storage areas for emotions. By toughening the fasciae and muscles, or by "freezing" the organs and intestines, the body can withhold emotions that you do not want to allow or deal with. Ask yourself: Which emotions do I tend to suppress or avoid alltogether? What are situations that make me hold my breath? When you consciously take a few deep breaths, you can help restore the flow of your emotions.

Between Sessions 5 and 6

Imagine, as you walk, that your legs do not begin at the hip joints but right below the ribs, in front of the lumbar spine. Visualize that, but do not consciously control or change the way you walk. Only observe what happens.

You can exercise your psoas muscles when you lie on your back, with your knees up. Gently roll your pelvis forward and back. Visualize how this movement originates from your lower back. This will help you move your pelvis from the inside, with the psoas muscle only. Keep your belly and pelvic floor muscles relaxed!

The Sixth Session

Body-Themes

In the sixth session, we focus on the core again, this time from the back. We try to establish good positioning of the pelvis and the sacrum. This usually includes work on the legs, as the best possible leg alignment is both a result and a prerequisite for a functioning pelvis-spine relation. Special emphasis will be placed on allowing the iliosacral joints (between sacrum and hip bone) to be stable as well as free to move properly. At this point, balancing the pelvis will cause the spine to lift up, relax and rest flexibly on top of the sacrum.

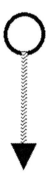

Fig. 14 A goal of the sixth session is to establish a resilient and alive connection between the sacrum and the head

Functionally, the goal of the sixth session is to establish fluidity in walking, with the legs being able to swing straight forward. The spine should be able to gently sway with movement and breathing and to retain its length as you walk, stand or pick something up. Furthermore, we include work to increase mobility in the hipjoints and iliosacral joints if necessary. We can also recheck the tone of the pelvic floor.

Psychological Themes

When you look in the mirror, you do not see your back. The back is what we do not normally show to the world; it is what we literally "keep back". Psychologically, our back harbors the dark sides of our personality, traits we often do not even want to acknowledge to ourselves. Take a moment to think about your dark sides. Can you look at them or are you trying to "keep them back"?

When we experience fear or anxiety, we tend to have our tailbone between our legs and to retract it by tightening our butt. When we do that, we close off true expression of self, power and creativity.

Between Sessions 6 and 7

Regardless of your breathing habits - whether you tend to belly-breathe or chest-breathe - try sending your breath into your upper and lower back a few times. This will allow you to breathe more deeply and relax your back. It will also help you establish contact with your emotions. Sometimes in life, you may feel overwhelmed by your emotions. In such situations, you can gain some clarity and objectivity when you make yourself aware of your breath filling the areas between your shoulderblades and around the thoracic spine.

The Seventh Session

Body-Themes

In the seventh session, lengthening and expanding core space are rounded off with work on the upper space of the core. The deep layers of the body, which have been balanced around the central vertical line in the previous sessions, provide the base for the head. The head should be able to balance on the neck with ease. So, session seven includes lengthening and repositioning of the neck and the head. Moreover, we will release the facial muscles, balance the joints of the jaw (TMJ's) and work on expanding the space inside the skull.

Easy, unrestricted and harmonious movement of neck, jaw and head are essential if we want to be perceptive of the world around us. Moreover, they will help our movements become more clearly directed and more flexible at the same time.

Psychological Themes

Session seven may take up the topic of the fourth session again: Am I clinging to things gritting my teeth or can I let go, too? "Keep smiling!" when I rather feel like clenching my teeth can give me an unconscious habit of teeth grinding at night.

Other issues you could explore are: Do I carry my head high, or do I walk through life as if it was weighing me down? Am I ducking from it alltogether? How does my head position affect the way I perceive my surroundings? How do I perceive the world around me? Do I narrow my perception down too much by focusing on immediate things only? Am I also able to notice what happens at the periphery? And, most important: Am I able to perceive myself perceiving?

Between Sessions 7 and 8

Visualize your head as a hot air balloon. Let it float upwards from your neck and allow it to be a natural extension of your spine. Do not pull your chin up or your neck back. Try that in standing, sitting and walking.

Imagine that your eyes are in the very center of your head, not at the front. Let the images come to you instead of staring hard at the world around you. You will not only be able to relax your vision but you will also help your head and neck stay well aligned.

When you do either of these exercises, remember: You are not trying to consciously change things. Instead, let the images do the work for you.

Sessions Eight and Nine

The last three sessions of the basic series provide the opportunity to bring all the newly organized structures and patterns into harmony with each other. The aim is to achieve integration, that is, to develop a balanced whole that is more than just the sum of all its parts.

We may, however, come back to some issues that we have worked with in the first seven sessions, this time emphasizing on how to best integrate them into the overall pattern.

Body-Themes

For both sessions, the aim is integration. However, in session eight we usually concentrate on the structure itself, whereas in session nine we tend to consider functional aspects more strongly. Session eight deals with overall structural stability, whereas session nine tries to establish balanced movement patterns.

A major element of this work is to establish horizontality of the shoulder and pelvic girdle (Fig. 15). Even more so than in the previous sessions, we consider the structural organization of the girdles in their relation with the core and the vertical inner line. We want them to connect well through the center of the body (Fig. 16). When we establish good balance and connection between the girdles and the inner space of the trunk, we are linking the center and periphery of your structure.

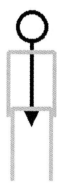

Fig. 15 Horizontal alignment of the pelvis girdle and the shoulder girdle

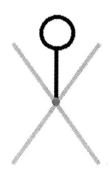

Fig. 16 Diagonal connection of the girdles through the body's core

One expression of such a good connection are more efficient patterns of arm and leg movement. The most important aspect of that is contralateral movement, which is visible when there is a funcional connection between each arm and the opposite leg. Moreover, we will finetune the coordination of intrinsic and extrinsic layers of musculature.

Psychological Themes

Core and inner vertical line are physical expressions of being, of the self. Shoulders, arms, pelvis and legs are physical expresssions of doing, of our activities in the world. Being and doing should be well balanced.

Look at yourself with this idea in mind: Do I tend to lose connection with my deep inner being, with myself, as I hustle through the activities of everyday life? Is my life based on my inner being or drifting with the changing forces around you? Do I listen to my inner voice telling me what is good and right for me? (you may also want to reconsider the psychological themes of sessions 2 and 3 here.)

Between Sessions 8, 9 and 10

Visualize your chest as a hot air balloon. Its center is right in the middle between your solar plexus (the place where the ribs meet the lower end of the sternum) and your spine. Your pelvis is the basket hanging from this hot air balloon. In standing or walking, visualize the hot air balloon of your chest floating upwards and the basket of your pelvis swinging freely underneath. Remember: never force it, just make the image vivid.

Take a walk and imagine your legs as moving from the center of the hot air balloon rather than from the hip joints.

If you want to work on allowing your arms to move more from your center, imagine that they begin in the area where the thoracic spine meets the lumbar spine rather than at the shoulders. Do your everyday arm-movements with this image in mind. Use this image also as you let your arms swing contralaterally when you walk.

If you want to relax your shoulder more when you lift your arm in front or at the side: Try letting your elbow and shoulder settle down as you breathe out (do not pull them down, only let them settle!). Finish this before you start lifting your arm to wherever you want. Make the movement slow, and ensure that your shoulder joint can stay open and relaxed. To feel the difference, make the same movement while you are consciously tightening the muscles in your shoulder area. Can you feel the difference? You can do this exercise many times in the course of a normal day, when you lift your coffee cup, pick up the phone, etc.

If you want to work on sitting some more, start with the sitting exercise I described after session one. The following suggestions will give you enough information to exhaustively explore and improve the way you sit.

1. Adjust the height of your chair (or find an appropriate one) so that your knees are just slightly below the level of your sitbones.

2. Make sure that at least one foot is positioned approximately under your knees or a little bit in front of it. If you pull your legs under or stretch them far out so that both feet are way in front or behind your knees, your knees will lack support and prevent the pelvis from finding a good position.

3. If your sitting position looks more like the lefthand drawing in Fig. 9 (p. 69), roll your pelvis forward until you hit the optimum forward-downward tilted position. Roll your pelvis around an imaginary side-to-side axis which rests on top of your hip joints. That is a little bit higher than the level of your groin fold. Roll the top of your hip bones forward over this axis until you feel yourself sitting in front of your sitbones. A lot of people are afraid that this may put them too much in a hollow back position. Do not worry about that. It will not, as long as you make sure your belly is relaxed and you do *not* use your low back muscles to roll your pelvis forward. Imagine that the front of your spine and the front of trunk and chest can lengthen upwards and downwards as you find this position.

4. If your upper back has a big curve (a tendency to hunch), your low back may still feel too tight. Try moving your entire trunk slightly forward from the

hipjoints. Do that slowly and gradually until you have reached a position where the tension in your low back is minimal and you feel you are balanced.

5. The weight of your trunk should now be *in front* of your hip joints and your trunk should rest effortlessly on top of your pelvis. That takes strain off your back and allows your neck and shoulder muscles to relax.

6. Very slight movements along the spine can save you from stiffening up when you sit and will keep you alert. Moreover, metabolic processes in the small muscles around the spine and the intervertebral joints will be enhanced. To allow these small motions, imagine your spine is a stalk of reedgrass or green bamboo, swaying gently with the breeze.

7. From the optimum sitting position, you can easily and without straining your back bend forward or down

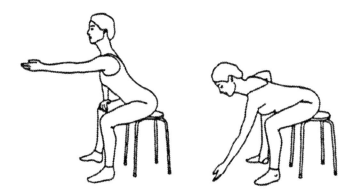

Fig. 17

(Fig. 17). Move from your hipjoints and allow your sitbones to glide backwards. Your belly should remain relaxed, so that your trunk can retain its slight convex curve in the front.

The Tenth Session

Body-Themes

The aim of the tenth session is to round off the integration process and provide closure. With that in mind, we again concentrate on two fundamental Rolfing goals: free movement of the joints and a flexible vertical body-axis which extends from the connection between thoracic and lumbar spine upwards and downwards.

Specifically, we want the client to be able to feel and be aware of the vertical inner line around which his/her body-structure organizes itself. Moreover, we focus once more on the horizontal balance of the paired joints (ankles, knees, hip joints, shoulders, elbows, wrists and jaw). Hallmarks of the complete integration of the organism are fluid and connected movements throughout the whole body.

Psychological Themes

When you look at somebody's joints you can get an impression of how mature they are. Stable, yet freely movable joints are characteristic of an adult person. Children's joints are still unstable, the joints of the elderly already somewhat stiff. This may reflect onto the psychological level, too. Being an adult means that your personality is stable but at the same time you are flexible enough to adapt to new situations. You are aware of your mental and physical limits and you can deal with them in a creative way. How do you experience yourself in this regard?

A body structure forms an integrated whole when all the body-segments relate to each other in a well-balanced and harmonious way. The same is true for our lives. Is there harmony in my life between thought, feeling and will? Many aspects together form a life: a loving relationship with a partner, children, work, recreation, friends, hobbies, spiritual life, etc. The amounts of time and energy spent on each should be well-balanced. Ideally, all areas of a life should relate to each other. Is part of my life separated off and alienated from the rest? Do some areas eat up all my energy while other needs are neglected?

You may have observed that as you progressed through your Rolfing series, you have become more aware of your own process and more willing to accept responsibility for it. You have become better able to handle this responsibility. The more you have come in contact with your inner self, the more you have experienced yourself as whole, yet structured. Being ready to take over responsibility for yourself and for your life - in a physical as well as in a emotional and spiritual sense - signifies maturity. Am I willing to take responsibility for my life? Do I use the freedom that comes with responsibility to be creative with my life?

After Session Ten

As you stand or walk, pay attention to the way your head is floating on top of your spine. Observe how your spine can relax a little when you allow your head to lift up just a bit more. As you feel this gentle (!) pull upwards through your head, make yourself aware of the slight downwards pull of gravity. You will feel gravity in the weight of your arms and shoulders, which should be resting on your trunk like a coat on its hanger.

Feel your inner line: It starts on the ground between your feet, comes up between your legs to the center of the pelvic floor, and continues along the front of your sacrum and spine to the crown of your head. Now visualize this line lengthening down into the ground and up into the sky. Do not force anything. Instead, feel and observe how you gain grounding and support as well as lightness and lift.

Observe yourself walking, be it indoor or outdoor: Where is your attention? Is it more within yourself, accompanied by habitually looking more downward to the ground? Try something else: Turn your perception (looking, listening, smelling) to the surrounding space. Perceive Nature, the houses and the people around you, feel the air, the sunshine or the rain on your skin and so forth. Summarizing said: Be aware of everything, which is in front of you (that is, where you are going to), of everything, which is beside you (that is, what is accompanying you), and of everything, which is behind you (that is, where you came from).

Being aware of your body sensations and the ground under your feet on the one hand, being attentive for your environment on the other hand - these are perceptions not necessarily excluding each other. Rather they complement and support each other, if you learn to let your mindfulness flow freely back and forth.

c. Open End

When the basic ten series of Rolfing is finished, it finishes with an open end. Your body will continue to process and integrate the impulses you have received during the sessions. As your improved body-structure is more at peace with gravity, the gravitational pull will support indirectly the process of integration and change. So, remain attentive to any changes that may occur on the physical or on other levels of life. Try to be aware of your body-mind. Listen to what it tells you. Your body will respond to all impulses, which may come from inside or outside.

Experiment with your new possibilities. It is a good idea to come back to this book now and then to go over the suggestions for each session again. Particularly the general section, but also the short passages on "psychological themes" and "between sessions" can be very helpful. Do not forget, though, that you should never doggedly work to improve your posture. The task is to playfully keep up with your body's evolution!

Although session 10 brings closure, you can of course continue your process with Rolfing. However, it is a good idea to observe a session-free integration period of approximately half a year. After that, you can take individual sessions to refresh your experience or continue deepening certain aspects of the work. If you need to regain your balance after a disruptive event like an accident, surgery or emotional trauma, Rolfing sessions will of course be helpful. Moreover, you can continue the work with *advanced Rolfing* sessions, which build on the results of the basic series and take them further onto a new level of complexive order.

Rolf Movement Integration, which is based on the same principles and goals as Rolfing Structural Integration, is another way to build on and develop the results of the basic series. Rolf Movement focuses on active perception and realizes change through an increase of awareness of

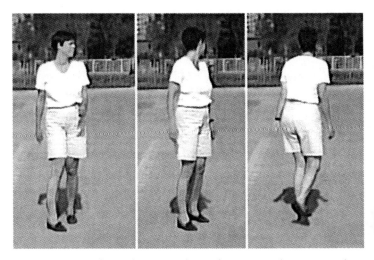

Fig. 18 Something from inside or from outside attracts the attention. The body follows this directional change of the attention through movement. Therefore movement is always an answer, is always a gesture.

structural and movement patterns as human expression (Fig. 18). The dominant aspect of this approach is movement rather than hands-on work. Rolf Movement is a great complement to Structural Integration. It is available through specifically trained *Rolf Movement Practitioners*.

If you want to continue exploring yourself moving, other approaches, such as *Structural Awareness* (similar to Rolf Movement), *Feldenkrais, Alexander Technique*, or disciplines like Aikido, Yoga or dance provide great opportunities too.

For further guidelines about self-improvement through movement practice, see recommended books on p. 113, written by *Mary Bond* and by *Alexandra and Roger Pierce*.

The next chapter will provide you with further suggestions for every day life.

4. Suggestions For Every Day Life

In this chapter I will make some practical suggestions which you can use in everyday life to support balance in your body structure. Naturally, these general suggestions cannot replace the individual devices of a Rolfer or Movement Practitioner. However, you can benefit from them even if you do not decide to get rolfed at this point in time.

a. Shoes - the Second Skin of Feet

Clothing is like a second skin to your body. This is especially important in the shoes you are wearing. Remember, your feet provide the foundation for your body-structure and therefore have significant influence on the quality of your movement. So, when you buy shoes, consider the following:

* The arches of your feet should always have enough space to compress and expand in a resilient way.
* Your shoes should be flexible enough not to impede the hinge-type movement between ankle and heel and between mid-foot and toes. Try walking in them for a few minutes before you buy.

* If the inner lining of your shoes pushes up on your inside arch, your weight will be brought over the outside edge of your foot. Such shoes are unsuitable.

* Soles and lining of your shoes should be flexible and allow your foot to adjust to various types of ground. Wooden soles, plateau shoes and the like prevent adaptive intrinsic foot movement.

* Sandals without straps across the heels force your toes to hold onto them. Continuous "clawing" like that will shorten muscles in the feet and will produce chronic tension in your calves.

* Shoes should allow you to easily pick up speed without abrupt, jerky muscle action. (Could you comfortably run for the bus in these shoes?)

* Negative heels (heels that are lower than the front part of the shoes) can be useful temporarily if your pelvis is structurally tilted too far forward and downward and the back of your legs is chronically short. This is common in people who have been wearing high heels for years.

b. About Sitting

Unfortunately, the optimum chair for the human structure has not yet been designed. Car seats tend to be among the worst. Most of their shapes tilt the pelvis backward so that you end up sitting on your tailbone rather than on your sitbones. This posture forestalls any lithe and supple body reaction and tends to produce neck pain, stiff shoulders and low pack pain.

How can you improve how you sit in your car? First of all, shift and tilt the seat so that the back approximates vertical and the seat is as horizontal as possible. A wedge-shaped support cushion under your buttocks can help your pelvis tilt forward properly and provide relief for your lower back. Watch your breathing and take care not to hold or constrict your breath. Keep your arms on the steering wheel and your legs as relaxed as possible.

In the sections on Rolfing-sessions one, eight and nine, I have discussed how to sit functionally and how important the correct height of your seat is. Here some additional tips:

When you read, write or work sitting at a table, make sure the height of the table fits the height of the chair *and* your own size. If the table is too high, resting the elbows or underarms on it will push your shoulders up. If the table is too low, you will tend to hunch your back. If your back has a tendency to hunch anyway, you may find it difficult to stay relaxed in an upright sitting posture. A wedge-shaped cushion can help. Also, whenever you have to sit for any length of time, take short breaks to bend forward, rest your chest on your thigh and relax arms and head like a resting coachman.

If you read a lot, you can avoid tensing your neck by bringing your book or magazine up into an oblique-vertical position in front of your eyes. This will allow your head and neck to stay in a more natural position instead of tilting them forward all the time. Bookrests or manuscript-stands from office supply stores are very useful here. There are even some height-adjustable book-stands available which allow you to read while relaxing into an armchair or on a couch.

c. Playful Exercise

Unfortunately, a lot of people seem to view sports as waging a war against their own bodies. They train themselves as if they were perfecting a machine to lose weight, build muscle or break a record. I would like to invite you to think of exercising in a more playful, more organic way. Cherish the intricacy of your movements and give them your attention. Playful exercise focuses on feeling good physically, on bringing balance to the system on all levels.

So, the most beneficial kinds of sports are those that work *all* the muscles *in a balanced way*. Swimming, hiking or cross-country skiing are good examples. Concentrating on a kind of sports that makes you use your body in a limited or one-sided way (like Tennis and muscle-training) stresses a very limited range of motions and will result in overspecialization. Because you over-use and over-develop certain body-parts and -functions at the expense of others. Your body will adapt to the lop-sided demand and develop structural imbalances which can, over time, wear out your joints and increase the risk of injury.

Moreover, muscle strengthening exercises like weights-lifting or body-building usually concentrate too much on developing the outer muscles and neglect the deep, inner muscles. Instead of opening from the inside and finding balance by finetuning the nervous system, your body can end up locked into a tight corset of fascial envelopes and your nervous system is not challenged in terms of proprioception. Since individual structural differences are not usually taken into account, these kinds of exercises tend to hide and reinforce structural imbalances.

If your everyday business does not include much movement at all, or if you tend to hold your emotions back, you may benefit most from interactive kinds of sports. Dance, martial arts or ball games provide lots of opportunity for expressive movement and human contact.

If you like to run, think about the following suggestions. They will help you develop better body-awareness and run in a more relaxed and efficient way. Of course, these ideas can be transferred to many other types of exercise. Be creative with them and explore rather that doggedly following the suggestions. Keep your sense of humor, be curious and loving with yourself and you will find that you improve much faster than with grim exercise.

* Run on unpaved ground. Running on pavement will expose your body to harsh impacts which it cannot cushion and absorb well.
* Are you holding your jaw? If yes, make sure you keep it relaxed and swingin'.

* Allow your facial muscles to relax. Your eyes should be gently gazing, not staring at things.

* Some runners tend to press their heads back and tighten the neck muscles. If you are doing that, bring your head into a more balanced position with your eyes horizontal and imagine it is a buoy floating on calm waters. Relax your neck and welcome the gentle bobbing movements to your head.

* Are you pressing your arms to your sides? Are you holding them in? Allow your arms to swing with the running motion. Your upper and lower arms can be more relaxed when you keep them at approximately a 90 degree angle. Avoid pulling the shoulders up or clenching your hands.

* If you are pushing your chest forward or drawing the shoulders back as you run, allow your breastbone to sink a little and let your shoulders sink slightly forward and down. If, on the other hand, your chest is collapsed and your shoulders are pulled forward, visualize an invisible thread that draws your breastbone slightly (!) up and to the front.

* Do not force your breath. Rather, allow the air to flow in and out. You can visualize your ribs floating on the river of your breath.

* Imagine that your pelvis is hanging from your chest like the basket of a hot air balloon.

* Some runners' legs seem to be dancing all over the place. (You can see that when you watch how feet

and knees move in relation to each other.) Imagine your knees are being pulled forward by invisible parallel strings. Another image you could visualize: your kneecaps lighting the space in front of you like the headlights on a car. These images will not only improve the straightforward motion of your knees, they will also have a positive influence on the way you transfer your weight from your heels over the balls of your feet with each step.

* When you explore running or other bodily activities with these suggestions in mind, perceive your movement entirely or stay in one area of your body for a while before shifting your attention. Focus on becoming aware of whatever your movement pattern is (even if it is problematic) before you try something new. Try going back and forth between old and new patterns a couple of times.

5. Sources

a. Addresses

Receive a list with *addresses* of Rolfers and Rolf Movement Practitioners and the *education guidelines* at these locations:

* **Rolf Institute of Structural Integration**
  205 Canyon Blvd.
  Boulder, CO 80302 (USA)
  phone: 303-449-5903
  e-mail: rolfinst@rolf.org
  web page: www.rolf.org

* **European Rolfing Association e.V.**
  Kapuzinerstrasse 25
  D - 80337 München (Germany)
  phone: 0049-89-54370941
  e-mail: rolfingeurope@compuserve.com
  web page: www.rolfing.org

* **Associacao Brasileira de Rolfistas**
  Caixa Postal 11299
  05422-970 Sao Paulo-SP (Brazil)
  phone: 011-55118870670
  e-mail: Rolfing@dialdata.com.br
  web page: www.rolfing.org.br

* **Australian Rolfing Office**
  90 Plateau Rd.
  Bilgola Plateau
  NSW Australia 2107
  phone: 011-61-02-99182324
  e-mail: JohnSmithSomatics@bigpond.com

Receive a list with *addresses* of Practitioners of Structural
Integration educated by the Guild for Structural Integration and the *education guidelines* at:

* **The Guild for Structural Integration**
  Post Office Box 1559
  Boulder, CO 80306 (USA)
  Phone: 303-447-0122
  e-mail: gsi@rolfguild.org
  web page: www.rolfguild.org

b. Recommended Books

Books on Rolfing and Structural Integration in general:

* *Ida P Rolf:* Rolfing. Reestablishing the Natural Alignment and Structural Integration of the Human Body for Vitality and Well-Being, Healing Arts Press 1989

   The standard reference about concept and method of Structural Integration.

* *Rosemary Feitis:* Ida Rolf Talks About Rolfing and Physical Reality, Harper and Row 1978

   The reader comes away with a vivid impression of Ida Rolf's thinking. The introduction by editor Rosemary Feitis presents details of Dr.Rolf's professional career.

* *Rosemary Feitis / Louis Schultz:* Remembering Ida Rolf, North Atlantic Books 1996

   A collection of stories about Ida Rolf. The book gives you a feeling for who she was and what she meant to her students.

* *Briah Anson:* Rolfing. Stories of Personal Empowerment, Heartland Personal Growth Press 1991

   This book is written from the point of view of persons who have been rolfed. Each of these experiences is unique and tells a story of physical and mental growth.

* *Mary Bond:* Balancing Your Body. A Self-Help Approach to Rolfing Movement, Healing Arts Press 1993

  Rolfer Mary Bond presents a self-help program of body transformation. The movement explorations are written as scripts so that you can practice the movements with detailed directions.

* *Alexandra* and *Roger Pierce*: Generous Movement. A practical Guide to Balance in Action, The Center of Balance Press 1991

  How can one find an easy balance in sitting, standing, walking, lifting, reaching in daily life? From the Rolfing perspective, the authors give a practical approach to such questions.

* *Brian W. Fahey:* The Power of Balance. A Rolfing View of Health, Metamorphous Press 1989

  Understanding how people organize their bodies to shape feeling, thought and behavior gives health professionals an avenue for helping clients improve their level of well-being.

Books on related topics:

* *Rosemary Feitis / Louis Schultz*: The Endless Web. Fascial Anatomy and Physical Reality, North Atlantic Books, 1996

A fully illustrated guide to understanding how the myofascia works, its suportive role within the body's anatomy, and how gentle manipulation of the myofascial tissue is central to lasting therapeutic intervention and how it can be integrated into any bodywork practice.

* *Louis Schultz:* Out in the Open. The Complete Male Pelvis,North Atlantic Books 1999

Combining many years of professional Rolfing experience with the precision of an academic anatomist, Louis Schultz examines the male pelvis under the dual lens of culture and science. A guide for bodyworkers and laypersons alike.

* *James L. Oschman:* Energy Medicine. The Scientific Basis, Churchill Livingstone 2000

What is the role of natural "energy forces" in the maintenance of health and wellbeing? Cell biologist James L. Oschman answers this question by bringing together evidence from a wide range of disciplines. The material presented is directly relevant to practitioners of a wide range of therapies.

* *Deane Juhan:* Job's Body, Station Hill Press 1987

Juhan provides an understanding of the mechanisms and effects of bodywork like Rolfing, Trager, Alexander, Feldenkrais etc. Furthermore, it can be read as a physiological textbook. Since it includes many facts, particularly about the nervous system and the connective tissue, which are hardly to find in academic medical textbooks.

* *Don Hanlon Johnson* (Ed.): Groundworks. Narratives of Embodiment, North Atlantic Books 1997

This book is a thoughtful account of how practitioners of various methods of bodywork (Lomi, Rolfing, Body-Mind Centering, Feldenkrais, Alexander etc.) actually go about the processes of working with individuals. It reveals the complexity of working with somatic processes.

* *Peter A.* Levine: Waking The Tiger, North Atlantic Books 1997

One of the world's leading experts in the field of trauma and stress offers a vision of healing trauma. Levine does not only help to understand the dynamics of trauma and trauma healing, rather the reader is enabled to employ a series of exercises that help to focus on bodily sensations, which is a step needed to heal trauma. A must for therapists and somatic practitioners as well as for persons affected.

* *Hans Georg Brecklinghaus:* The Human Beings are awoken, you have set them upright. Body Structure and Conception of Man in Ancient Egyptian Art and The Present Day (forthcoming book)

Through examples and by comparison with other ancient civilizations, the author illustrates how ancient Egyptian portrayals of man demonstrate a well integrated body structure and economic movement patterns. It becomes obvious that the artists and craftsmen in ancient Egypt were primarily inspired by their old culture's conception of Human Being. Furthermore, the author shows how a deeper understanding of these aspects of ancient Egyptian art can be of value for present day man.

* *Erick Hawkins:* The Body Is A Clear Place. And Other Statements On Dance, Dance Horizons Books, 1992

  The book is a collection of essays that serve as a testament to Erick Hawkins' long career in dance. It challenges us to revolutionize our responses to movement and dance. Hawkins has created an aesthetic of movement based on a clear understanding of the science of movement. Hawkins' notion is that art can exist both for its own sake and as a means toward deeper enlightenment.

Illustrations Citation Index

Hans Georg Brecklinghaus (3, 5, 6, 7, 14, 15, 16, 17, 18)
Hans Flury (4)
Hummel (8, 10, 11)
Carlos Repetto (2, 9, 12, 13)
Rolf Institute of Struetural Integration, Boulder (CO) (1)

Note: Publisher and author tried to find the holder of the copyright of the original of the cover illustration, but without success. Provided that the holder informs us about his/her rights we shall indicate him/her as such.

Another forthcoming book of the same author:

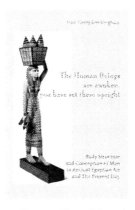

Hans Georg Brecklinghaus

The Human Beings are awoken, you have set them upright

Body Structure and Conception of Man
in Ancient Egyptian Art and The Present Day

338 pp., 109 Fig.   ISBN 3-932803-04-3

In this book, the author illustrates that Egyptian artistic portrayals of man present a well integrated body structure and economical movement patterns.

Egyptian artists and craftsmen were primarily inspired by their old culture's conception of life and of man.

It is made apparent that both aspects of ancient Egyptian art, the exemplary movement presented and a specific spiritual view of life, can be of value for present day human being.